Autism at 30, 40, 50

Real Stories of Late Diagnosis Across the
Decades and the Life That Follows

Vionnet Vilina McKinney

The stories shared in " Autism at 30, 40, 50: Real Stories of Late Diagnosis Across the Decades and the Life That Follows" are composites drawn from the authentic, lived experiences of numerous individuals. These narratives reflect common themes, challenges, and triumphs reported by late-identified autistic people across various demographics and backgrounds. While each story is rooted in real accounts and aims to be representative, they are not direct, one-to-one portrayals of any single individual. Details have been altered, combined, or condensed to protect privacy, illustrate key points effectively, and ensure broad relatability. **Any resemblance to specific persons, living or deceased, is purely coincidental.**

This book is intended to provide information, understanding, and a sense of community for readers. It is not a substitute for professional medical, psychological, or diagnostic advice. If you suspect you or someone you know may be autistic, or if you are seeking support for mental health challenges, please consult with a qualified healthcare professional. The resources provided in this book are for informational purposes only and should not be considered an endorsement or a definitive list of all available services.

ISBN: 978-1-7641941-1-2
Isohan Publishing

Table of Contents

Introduction

Late autism identification has quietly shaped many lives. For years, countless individuals have moved through the world with an underlying sense of disconnect, a feeling that they don't quite fit the mold everyone else seems to occupy. This book pulls back the curtain on these private experiences, offering a collection of stories from those who, later in life, came to understand themselves through the lens of autism. Our purpose here is simple: to share these diverse lived experiences, to illuminate common threads, and to create a space of recognition and connection for anyone who has felt that persistent "something's different" nagging at them. When we talk about "late-identified autism," we are including both those who received a formal "diagnosis" and those who, through careful introspection and community engagement, have "identified" as autistic. The invitation to you, the reader, is straightforward: if any of these stories echo your own quiet questions, know this – you are not alone.

Chapter 1: The Lingering Question

Many individuals live for decades with an unspoken question hanging over their heads: **Why do I feel so fundamentally different?** It's a question that doesn't often find voice because, without a framework for understanding, it remains a diffuse, unsettling sensation. This feeling can manifest as persistent social struggles, overwhelming sensory sensitivities, chronic burnout, and an overall sense that the "rules" of life are just a bit different for them than for everyone else. Often, these feelings are managed through **masking**, a term for consciously or unconsciously hiding or camouflaging autistic traits to fit in, and **compensatory strategies**, which are learned behaviors to navigate social or sensory challenges. The effort involved in this can be immense, leading to profound exhaustion and a deep-seated feeling that they are constantly performing, never truly themselves.

Consider Sarah, a woman in her late 40s [1]. From childhood, Sarah felt like an alien observing human interactions. She'd spend hours analyzing conversations, trying to decipher unspoken cues, yet often missed obvious social jokes. Her teachers praised her for being "quiet and studious," but she recalled the sheer terror of group projects, where the unwritten social hierarchy and spontaneous chitchat felt like a foreign language. Loud noises, strong perfumes, and scratchy clothes were not just annoying; they were physically painful, often sending her into a state of agitated overwhelm she couldn't explain. She developed a complex system of internal rules for social situations, like "smile and nod when people talk about the weather" or "ask three questions about the other person before talking about yourself." These were her compensatory strategies, her carefully constructed shield. The problem was, maintaining this shield was utterly draining. By the time she got home from work, she'd often collapse, unable to speak or interact, leading to friction with her family who saw her as moody or disengaged. She always felt like she was trying to solve a puzzle with missing pieces, constantly questioning her own perceptions and reactions. She'd wonder, "Why does everyone else seem to manage this so easily?" This internal query, a persistent, low hum of uncertainty, followed her for decades.

Another example is Michael, a man in his early 50s who, despite a successful career in engineering, always felt out of sync with his colleagues [2]. He excelled at his technical work, able to focus intently on complex problems for hours without distraction. However, team meetings were a source of dread. He struggled with small talk, often finding himself staring at people's shoes or the clock, desperate for the conversation to shift back to concrete tasks. He found the fluorescent lights and constant hum of the office deeply unsettling, often wearing noise-canceling headphones even when not on calls, which some colleagues perceived as rude. Michael learned to nod along in conversations, offering generic affirmations like "That's interesting" or "I see," hoping to appear engaged. He meticulously prepared for any social event, mentally scripting conversations and planning his escape routes. This constant self-monitoring, the effort of maintaining his "normal" facade, was exhausting. He often felt a profound sense of loneliness, despite being surrounded by people, because he couldn't truly express his authentic self. The "lingering question" for Michael was why social interactions felt like such an arduous performance rather than a natural flow.

Then there is Clara, a woman in her late 30s who, for years, attributed her chronic fatigue and anxiety to her demanding job [3]. She was known for her intense focus on details and her preference for working alone. However, sudden changes in routine at work or unexpected social invitations would send her into a spiral of internal panic. She often found herself unable to filter out background noise, making it almost impossible to concentrate in open-plan offices. Clara developed a strong ability to mimic social cues she observed in others, effectively creating a highly convincing "social persona." She'd rehearse conversations in her head, practice facial expressions in the mirror, and even research popular culture topics to have something to talk about. This **masking** was so effective that most people considered her "charming" and "outgoing." Yet, beneath this polished exterior, Clara was in constant distress. She suffered from unexplained stomach issues and frequent migraines, which doctors struggled to diagnose. She always felt like she was playing a part, never truly relaxed, wondering why her internal experience of life seemed so much more effortful and overwhelming than that of her peers. The quiet, nagging question for Clara was, "Why does being me feel so hard?"

These are just a few glimpses into the world of individuals living with the lingering question of undiagnosed autism. The common thread is the immense, often invisible, effort of navigating a world not designed for their neurology. The burnout isn't just physical; it's a deep, existential exhaustion born from the continuous act of camouflaging one's true self. They are not simply "shy" or "awkward"; they are processing the world differently, experiencing it with a unique set of sensitivities, and often, without understanding why. This lack of understanding can lead to self-blame, feelings of inadequacy, and a profound sense of isolation.

Key Takeaways

- **Undiagnosed individuals often feel fundamentally different**, leading to persistent questions about their internal experiences.

- **Masking and compensatory strategies** are common ways people manage these differences, but they lead to significant **burnout and exhaustion**.

- The effort of fitting in can result in **chronic stress, anxiety, and physical symptoms** that are difficult to explain.

- This feeling of being "out of sync" often leads to **self-blame and isolation**, as they lack a framework for understanding their experiences.

Chapter 2: The Childhood Reimagined

For many late-identified autistic individuals, receiving an autism explanation later in life isn't just about understanding their present struggles; it's a profound re-reading of their entire past. **Childhood memories**, once seen as quirks, social missteps, or unexplained anxieties, suddenly click into place. The **"aha!" moments** flood in, creating a powerful sense of clarity about behaviors and experiences that previously made no sense. It's like finding the legend to a map they've been trying to navigate blindly for decades. This reinterpretation isn't about changing the past, but about understanding it with new eyes, forgiving past perceived "failures," and recognizing the true nature of their early existence.

Take the case of David, a man in his 50s, who always considered himself an "odd kid" [4]. His parents often recounted stories of his intense interests – collecting and categorizing every type of rock he could find, meticulously organizing his comic book collection by publication date and artist, and spending hours dismantling and reassembling electronics. While others played sports, David preferred to sit alone, drawing intricate schematics or reading encyclopedias. Socially, he remembered feeling perpetually confused. Playtime on the schoolyard felt chaotic; he didn't understand the complex rules of playground games or the constant shifts in alliances among his peers. He preferred the predictability of solitary play, which led to him being labeled "a loner." He'd often get overwhelmed by the noise of the classroom or the smell of the cafeteria, leading to meltdowns that were dismissed as "tantrums" or "being oversensitive." After his autism explanation at 52, David revisited these memories. The intense interests weren't just hobbies; they were **special interests** – deep, passionate dives into specific topics. His discomfort with social games wasn't shyness; it was a genuine difficulty with social cues and unstructured play. His meltdowns were **sensory overload** and **autistic shutdowns**, not tantrums. This reinterpretation brought a wave of both sadness for what he didn't know and immense relief, as his past finally made sense.

Consider Eleanor, a woman in her early 60s who struggled academically in primary school despite being highly intelligent [5]. Her teachers often complained about her "lack of focus" and her tendency to stare out the window. What they didn't realize was that Eleanor was overwhelmed by the buzzing of the fluorescent lights, the scratch of chalk on the blackboard, and the constant movement of other children. She found it hard to filter out these distractions, making it almost impossible to concentrate on lessons. She was also a literal thinker; when a teacher told her to "pull herself together," she'd literally try to physically gather herself, leading to confusion. She preferred quiet activities, like reading for hours or sketching detailed drawings of animals. Socially, she often felt excluded. She didn't understand why other girls would whisper secrets or form cliques. Her attempts to join groups often ended in awkwardness, as she would offer facts rather than engage in casual banter. After her autism explanation, Eleanor realized her "lack of focus" was **sensory distraction** and **autistic inertia**, her literal interpretation of language a common autistic trait. Her preference for solitary pursuits was not anti-social behavior but a need for **low-demand environments** and the deep satisfaction of her **special**

7

interests. She understood why she felt so exhausted after school – it was the constant effort of trying to process an overwhelming environment and decipher unwritten social rules.

Then there's Leo, a man in his 40s, who was diagnosed with ADHD in childhood, which partially explained some of his difficulties, but never fully captured his experience [6]. He was known for his boundless energy and rapid shifts between interests, but also for his rigid routines and extreme distress when those routines were disrupted. He recalled intense fixations on specific topics, like trains or dinosaurs, which he would talk about endlessly, often to the discomfort of his peers. Socially, he was often seen as "blunt" or "tactless" because he would state facts directly without sugarcoating them or considering the social implications. He found eye contact painful and avoided it, which was often misinterpreted as disinterest or rudeness. When Leo received his autism explanation in his late 30s, his "ADHD" was recontextualized. His intense fixations were classic **autistic special interests**. His need for routine and distress at change were manifestations of **autistic rigidity and a need for predictability**. His "bluntness" was not malice but a difference in communication style, often called **"autistic directness."** The discomfort with eye contact was a common **sensory difference**. The ADHD was still there, but autism provided the missing pieces, allowing him to understand the underlying reasons for so many of his childhood struggles and "failures."

These examples show how a later understanding of autism can completely **transform one's narrative of childhood**. It shifts the perspective from "I was a difficult child" or "I just didn't try hard enough" to "I was an autistic child navigating a world not set up for my brain." This reinterpretation is not just academic; it's deeply healing. It allows individuals to shed years of self-blame, shame, and confusion, replacing them with self-compassion and a clearer understanding of their own unique operating system. It illuminates the sheer resilience they displayed in adapting and surviving without the proper tools or explanations.

Key Takeaways

- **Late autism identification leads to a reinterpretation of childhood memories**, providing clarity and understanding.

- Childhood behaviors, once seen as oddities or failures, are recognized as **autistic traits or responses to an unaccommodating environment.**

- This reinterpretation helps individuals **shed self-blame** and develop self-compassion for their past experiences.

- Understanding their early life through an autistic lens reveals their **inherent resilience** in navigating a world without proper understanding or support.

Chapter 3: Navigating Relationships and Society

Relationships, in all their varied forms – friendships, romantic partnerships, family dynamics – present a complex maze for many, particularly for those who are later identified as autistic. Before understanding their autistic neurology, individuals often wrestle with **challenges in communication, emotional regulation, and a persistent feeling of being an outsider in social settings**. This leads to misunderstandings, hurt feelings, and a profound sense of loneliness, even when surrounded by people. The invisible "manual" of social interaction seems to be missing for them, leaving them to guess, mimic, and often, miss the mark.

Consider Alex, a non-binary individual in their early 30s [7]. Alex consistently struggled with friendships, often feeling like they were playing a role rather than being genuinely connected. They found **small talk** excruciating, preferring to discuss deep, specific interests, which sometimes led to others perceiving them as intense or awkward. Alex also found it difficult to understand **unspoken social rules** – when to text, how long to wait to reply, or the nuances of sarcasm and irony. They often took things literally, leading to misinterpretations and unintended offense. For example, a casual invitation to "hang out sometime" would be taken as a firm commitment, leading to confusion when no specific plans materialized. In romantic relationships, Alex found the emotional intensity overwhelming. They struggled with **identifying and articulating their own emotions**, often feeling a surge of undifferentiated distress rather than distinct anger or sadness. This made conflict resolution particularly difficult, as they couldn't easily explain what they were feeling or needing. They often felt like an outsider looking in, observing others navigate social spaces with an effortless grace that eluded them.

Another example is Ben, a man in his late 40s, who, despite having a long-term marriage, often felt a profound disconnect from his wife and children [8]. He struggled with what his wife called his "lack of empathy" – he found it hard to instinctively respond to her emotional cues or to offer comfort in the way she expected. For instance, when his wife was upset about a work issue, Ben would immediately offer logical solutions rather than validating her feelings, which often made her feel unheard. He found family gatherings overwhelming due to the noise, the unstructured conversation, and the constant demands for eye contact. He would often retreat to a quiet room, which was perceived as being antisocial or disinterested. Ben's **communication style was very direct**, leading to friction when he unknowingly offended someone. He also had a hard time with unexpected changes to plans, which were frequent in his busy family life, leading to meltdowns or shutdowns he couldn't explain to them. He often wondered why he couldn't just "be normal" and connect with his loved ones in the way he saw others do. This sense of being an **outsider** within his own family was a heavy burden.

Then there's Chloe, a woman in her mid-30s, who maintained a small but loyal group of friends, yet struggled with the unspoken expectations of group dynamics [9]. She often found herself accidentally interrupting others or monopolizing conversations when discussing her special interests. She had difficulty processing multiple conversations at once, often zoning out in noisy social settings. Chloe also found the concept of "flirting" baffling, often missing romantic cues entirely or misinterpreting platonic gestures. She struggled with **emotional regulation**, particularly when overwhelmed, leading to intense meltdowns that she would later feel immense shame about. These incidents often left her feeling isolated, believing there was something fundamentally "wrong" with her ability to connect. For example, an unexpected change of plans for a weekend trip with friends might trigger intense anxiety and irritability, which her friends perceived as her being "difficult" rather than understanding it as a response to a disrupted routine and the resulting sensory overload. She spent years trying to decode the "rules" of friendship, often leading to overthinking every social interaction and feeling exhausted by the effort.

These narratives highlight the profound impact of undiagnosed autism on social and relational well-being. The **challenges with communication** aren't a lack of desire to connect, but often a difference in how information is processed and expressed. **Emotional regulation** difficulties stem from an often overwhelming internal experience of emotions and difficulty processing sensory input, leading to shutdowns or meltdowns when the system is overloaded. The persistent feeling of being an **outsider** is a direct result of navigating a neurotypical-centric social world without the inherent understanding of its unwritten rules. These experiences often lead to chronic feelings of loneliness, misunderstanding, and a deep yearning for genuine connection that feels just out of reach.

Key Takeaways

- **Undiagnosed autism often leads to difficulties in social communication and emotional regulation** within relationships.

- Individuals may struggle with **unspoken social rules, literal interpretation, and sensory overwhelm** in social settings.

- This can result in feelings of **being an outsider, misunderstanding, and profound loneliness**.

- The effort to navigate these challenges often leads to **exhaustion and self-blame**, impacting their ability to form deep connections.

Chapter 4: The Professional Mask

For many late-identified autistic individuals, the workplace becomes a grand stage where they hone their **professional mask**. This isn't just about presenting a polished image; it's about meticulously suppressing autistic traits and adopting compensatory behaviors to fit into neurotypical corporate structures. The effort required for this can be immense, leading to **career changes, job hopping, and severe burnout**. The constant pressure to conform, to engage in small talk, to navigate unspoken office politics, and to manage sensory input in often overwhelming environments creates an unsustainable level of stress, all before understanding their underlying needs.

Consider Elena, a woman in her early 60s, who had a string of administrative roles throughout her career [10]. Elena was incredibly organized, meticulous, and reliable, excelling in tasks that required attention to detail and adherence to process. However, she struggled immensely with office politics and social dynamics. She found team-building exercises excruciating, often preferring to eat lunch alone at her desk rather than engage in forced conversation. She was often misunderstood as "cold" or "aloof" because she struggled to make eye contact or engage in casual chitchat. Elena found open-plan offices a sensory nightmare – the constant chatter, phone calls, and background noise made it impossible for her to concentrate, leading to frequent headaches and irritability. To cope, she developed a **highly rigid routine** at work, which helped her manage sensory input and unpredictable social interactions. Any deviation from this routine, like an unexpected meeting or a last-minute project, would cause extreme stress and overwhelm.

She experienced frequent burnout, leading her to "job hop" every few years, always seeking a quieter environment or a role with less social interaction, never quite understanding why each new job eventually led to the same exhaustion.

Another example is Robert, a man in his mid-50s, a brilliant software engineer who was often lauded for his technical prowess but criticized for his "poor communication skills" [11]. Robert could spend hours coding, deeply engrossed in complex problems. However, he struggled with presentations, feeling overwhelmed by the pressure of public speaking and the need to read a room. He often spoke in a monotone voice and struggled to modulate his tone, which was sometimes perceived as disinterest or rudeness. He also had a strong **preference for direct communication** and found indirect or implied requests confusing and frustrating. For example, if a manager hinted at a problem without explicitly stating it, Robert would miss the cue entirely. He often found himself misunderstood in meetings, where his literal interpretations of instructions or questions led to miscommunications. Robert frequently experienced **sensory overload** from the bright office lights and the constant chatter of his colleagues, leading him to retreat to quiet corners or work late into the night when the office was empty. This constant effort to translate his thoughts into neurotypical communication styles and to manage sensory input led to frequent burnout, making him question his own competence despite his clear technical abilities. He often felt a deep sense of frustration, wondering why others found this seemingly effortless.

Then there's Maria, a woman in her 40s, who excelled in creative roles but struggled with the constant demand for networking and self-promotion [12]. Maria was a talented graphic designer, able to conceptualize unique visual solutions and produce stunning work with meticulous detail. However, industry events, client presentations, and even casual team brainstorming sessions filled her with dread. She found it difficult to generate spontaneous ideas in group settings and often felt overwhelmed by the unwritten rules of networking – who to approach, what to say, how to make small talk. She learned to **mask her discomfort** by rehearsing polite phrases and forcing herself to make eye contact, even though it was physically painful. Maria also had a **strong need for predictability** and found the ever-changing demands of creative projects highly stressful. She would often work long hours, pushing herself to the brink of exhaustion to meet deadlines, driven by a fear of failure and a need for control over her output. She experienced multiple periods of severe burnout, leading her to take extended breaks or even consider leaving her profession entirely, attributing her struggles to a "lack of resilience" rather than an unrecognized neurotype. The professional mask she wore was so convincing that no one suspected the immense internal struggle.

These stories illustrate the profound cost of **masking in the workplace**. The professional mask, while often enabling individuals to maintain employment, comes at a severe personal expense. The energy expended to suppress natural autistic traits, to mimic neurotypical social behaviors, and to tolerate overwhelming sensory environments leads to chronic stress, anxiety, and **significant burnout**. This cycle of pushing through, burning out, and then searching for a new environment often perpetuates until the underlying reason for these struggles – autism – is finally understood. The "effort expended to conform" is not a minor inconvenience; it is a fundamental drain on an individual's life force, impacting their well-being far beyond the confines of the office.

Key Takeaways

- **Many late-identified autistic individuals develop a "professional mask" to conform** in the workplace.

- This masking involves **suppressing autistic traits and adopting compensatory behaviors**, leading to significant exhaustion.

- Workplace challenges include **social dynamics, sensory overwhelm, and communication differences**, often resulting in burnout and job changes.

- The constant effort to fit in can obscure **underlying autistic needs**, leading to self-blame and a cycle of career dissatisfaction.

Chapter 5: The Search for Answers (and Misdiagnoses)

Before an autism explanation comes to light, many individuals embark on a protracted and often frustrating journey through various medical and psychological systems, seeking an explanation for their pervasive difficulties. This often leads to a series of **misdiagnoses**, where symptoms are attributed to other conditions like anxiety, depression, or personality disorders. This cycle of seeking help, receiving an incomplete or inaccurate diagnosis, and experiencing ongoing struggles takes a significant **emotional toll**, leaving individuals feeling misunderstood, invalidated, and increasingly hopeless about finding a path to well-being.

Consider Daniel, a man in his early 20s, who had been in therapy since his late teens for what was primarily diagnosed as **generalized anxiety disorder** and **social anxiety** [13]. He reported persistent worry, difficulty initiating conversations, and an overwhelming fear of judgment in social situations. However, his anxiety treatments never quite seemed to stick. While therapists focused on cognitive restructuring and exposure therapy, Daniel found that his anxiety wasn't just about "irrational thoughts." It was rooted in an inability to understand social cues, a deep discomfort with eye contact, and an overwhelming sensory experience of crowded spaces. He'd try to push himself into social situations, as advised, but would often end up in a state of meltdown or shutdown, which his therapists interpreted as "panic attacks" or "avoidant behavior." He was also prescribed various medications for anxiety, which offered limited relief. The constant cycle of trying, failing, and feeling misunderstood led to a profound sense of despair, making him question if he was simply "untreatable." His experience exemplifies how autistic traits, when not recognized, can be mistaken for other mental health conditions, leading to ineffective interventions and prolonged suffering.

Another example is Olivia, a woman in her mid-30s, who had been diagnosed with **Borderline Personality Disorder (BPD)** in her late 20s after years of intense emotional dysregulation, unstable relationships, and impulsivity [14]. She experienced extreme mood swings, often going from calm to intense anger or despair in a short period. Her relationships were characterized by cycles of idealization and devaluation, and she struggled with a pervasive feeling of emptiness. While some aspects of BPD seemed to fit, Olivia always felt that the diagnosis missed something crucial. Her "emotional dysregulation" was often triggered by sensory overload or unexpected changes, leading to meltdowns that were interpreted as "splitting." Her struggles with relationships stemmed not from a fear of abandonment (though that was present), but from a genuine difficulty in understanding social nuances, communicating her needs, and processing complex social interactions. Her "impulsivity" sometimes manifested as extreme reactions to perceived injustices or rigid adherence to rules, which didn't quite fit the typical BPD narrative. The BPD label often led to her feeling pathologized and misunderstood, with therapists focusing on her "manipulative" behaviors rather than the underlying distress caused by unrecognized autistic traits. The emotional toll of this misdiagnosis was immense, leading to self-stigma and a sense that she was fundamentally flawed.

Then there is Paul, a man in his 50s, who, after a lifetime of feeling "off," eventually received a diagnosis of **Obsessive-**

Compulsive Personality Disorder (OCPD) [15]. He was known for his extreme perfectionism, rigid adherence to rules, and difficulty delegating tasks. He had routines he adhered to with unwavering precision, and any deviation caused him significant distress. While OCPD accounted for some of these behaviors, it didn't explain his intense sensory sensitivities (e.g., to certain textures or sounds), his literal interpretation of language, or his social awkwardness. Paul also experienced deep internal anxiety and exhaustion from the constant effort of maintaining his routines and trying to control his environment, which went beyond typical OCPD traits. For instance, his need for objects to be arranged in a specific way wasn't just about orderliness; it was a way to manage sensory input and reduce cognitive load. The misdiagnosis led therapists to focus on "reducing his rigidity" without understanding that these behaviors were often his coping mechanisms for an overwhelming world. He felt like his core struggles were being dismissed or misinterpreted, leaving him stuck in a loop of ineffective treatments and continued internal suffering.

These detailed examples lay bare the profound impact of **misdiagnoses** on late-identified autistic individuals. The "search for answers" becomes a bewildering and disheartening maze, where their genuine struggles are frequently misinterpreted through the lens of conditions that don't fully capture their unique neurotype. The "emotional toll" is heavy, leading to prolonged distress, self-blame, and a sense of alienation from the very systems designed to help. Without the correct explanation, these individuals are left to navigate a world that makes little sense to them, constantly battling internal and external misunderstandings, and feeling that true well-being is an elusive dream.

Key Takeaways

- **Many late-identified autistic individuals endure years of misdiagnoses** for conditions like anxiety, depression, or personality disorders.

- This cycle of incorrect explanations leads to **ineffective treatments and prolonged suffering**.

- The **emotional toll is significant**, fostering feelings of invalidation, hopelessness, and self-blame.

- Without an accurate understanding of autism, individuals remain stuck in a **perpetual search for answers**, unable to address their true needs.

Final Reflections

The narratives shared in these initial pages offer a window into the lived experiences of individuals before the clarity of late autism identification. They paint a picture of quiet struggle, persistent questions, and the immense, often invisible, effort of navigating a world that doesn't quite fit. From the lingering sense of being an outsider, to the reinterpretation of childhood memories, the challenges of social navigation, the strain of the professional mask, and the frustrating journey through misdiagnoses – these stories reveal a common thread: the profound cost of not knowing oneself. Yet, even within these struggles, we see incredible resilience and an enduring spirit. These individuals have, in their own ways, forged paths through confusion, demonstrating a remarkable capacity to adapt and survive. As we move forward, we will witness the transformative power of self-understanding and the profound relief that comes with finally answering that persistent question: "Why do I feel so fundamentally different?"

Chapter 6: The "Aha!" Moment

The moment of realizing one might be autistic, often decades into life, can hit like a lightning bolt. It's not always a dramatic event; sometimes it's a quiet whisper that grows louder until it can't be ignored. These **specific triggers** range widely, but they all share one thing: they connect previously disparate experiences under a single, unifying explanation. This realization brings with it a complex mix of feelings. There's often an initial **shock**, as the idea challenges a lifetime of self-perception. But almost immediately, this shock is followed by immense **relief** – a profound sense that they aren't "broken" or "wrong," but simply wired differently. This is then coupled with powerful **validation**, as years of struggle and misunderstanding finally have a name.

Consider Frank, a man in his 40s [16]. Frank had always felt like an outsider. He was good at his engineering job (precise, logical), but social events exhausted him. He'd spend hours replaying conversations, trying to figure out what he'd missed. One evening, his long-time friend, Sarah, told him she had just received an autism explanation. As Sarah described her experiences – her sensitivity to fluorescent lights, her difficulty with small talk, her need for rigid routines, and her tendency to take things literally – Frank felt a jolt. "That sounds exactly like me," he thought. He listened intently as Sarah talked about masking, about the sheer exhaustion of pretending to be "normal." He went home that night and searched for information about adult autism. Every checklist, every personal account, felt like reading his own biography. The trigger was Sarah's experience, which acted as a mirror. The initial shock quickly gave way to a powerful sense of **relief**. "It wasn't me being bad at people," he told himself. "It was just a different operating system." The **validation** was immediate; suddenly, his entire life of feeling "off" had a reason. He wasn't failing; he was simply processing the world in a way others didn't.

Another example is Emily, a woman in her late 30s who stumbled upon her "aha!" moment through social media [17]. Emily had always been labeled "shy" and "anxious." She found loud environments overwhelming and preferred to spend her free time researching obscure historical topics. She had a small group of trusted friends, but often felt drained after social outings, even with them. One day, while scrolling through a popular video platform, she saw a short clip of an autistic woman describing her sensory sensitivities and how she "stimmed" (self-stimulatory behaviors like fidgeting or rocking) to cope. Emily watched, mesmerized, as the woman described feeling overwhelmed by bright lights and strong smells, and how she'd retreat to quiet spaces to "recharge." Emily had always bitten the inside of her cheek when stressed, a habit she thought was just a nervous tic. The video also touched on **special interests** and **autistic burnout**. As Emily watched more videos by autistic creators, she realized that so many of their shared experiences – from specific sensory issues to communication styles – mirrored her own. The trigger was a simple TikTok video that brought her into contact with autistic voices. The **initial shock** of thinking she might be autistic was quickly followed by an outpouring of tears – tears of **relief** that she finally understood herself. It was as if a lifelong weight had been lifted, replaced by a profound sense of **validation** that her experiences were real and shared.

Then there is Carlos, a man in his 50s, whose "aha!" moment came from reading a book [18]. Carlos had always been a quiet observer, preferring solitary activities like woodworking or tending to his extensive garden. He prided himself on his logical thinking but often found human emotions bewildering. His wife frequently complained that he was "too literal" and "didn't listen" when she expressed feelings. He had a meticulous approach to his hobbies, where precision and order were paramount. One day, his daughter, a psychology student, recommended a book about adult neurodiversity. Carlos, ever curious, began reading it. As he read descriptions of individuals who struggled with unspoken social rules, had a need for routine, and experienced sensory overload, he felt an uncanny recognition. The book talked about "theory of mind" challenges and how autistic people might struggle to intuit others' thoughts or feelings. Carlos had always wondered why social interactions felt like a complex equation he was constantly trying to solve. The trigger was the book, offering a structured way to understand his own experiences. The **shock** was immediate – "Could this be me?" he wondered. But as he continued reading, a profound **relief** washed over him. The book described the common autistic trait of difficulty with "emotional empathy" while often having strong "cognitive empathy" (the ability to logically understand another person's perspective). This explained his wife's complaints. The **validation** was immense; it explained his literalness, his intense focus on hobbies, and his social struggles. He felt like he had been living in a foggy room his whole life, and suddenly, someone had turned on the light.

These stories illustrate that the **"aha!" moment** is rarely a gentle realization; it is often an emotionally charged event. It's the sudden clarity that connects disparate pieces of a life, leading to an immediate sense of relief that the struggle has a name and a context. This powerful validation allows individuals to begin shedding years of self-blame and to step onto a path of self-acceptance and understanding. The journey from this moment onward is about re-evaluating everything that came before with new eyes.

Key Takeaways

- The **"aha!" moment** is a sudden, often emotional, realization of autistic identity.

- It's typically triggered by **specific external factors** like a friend's explanation, social media content, or a book.

- Initial feelings include **shock and disbelief**, quickly followed by immense **relief and validation**.

- This understanding provides a **framework for past struggles**, replacing self-blame with self-compassion.

Chapter 7: The Diagnostic Journey

Once the "aha!" moment hits, many individuals choose to pursue a **formal diagnosis**. This journey, however, is rarely straightforward. It often presents significant **challenges**, including facing skepticism from medical professionals, navigating long waiting lists, and encountering **gender bias** in diagnostic criteria. The process can be emotionally taxing, yet for many, the **profound impact of finally receiving official confirmation** makes every hurdle worthwhile. It provides not just a label, but often access to support, a sense of belonging, and a powerful validation of their reality.

Take the story of Grace, a woman in her early 30s [19]. After her "aha!" moment, Grace started researching diagnostic services. She quickly found that adult autism diagnostic pathways were limited and often had **waiting lists stretching for years** in her area. When she finally secured an appointment with a private psychologist, she faced initial **skepticism**. The psychologist noted that Grace made good eye contact (a learned skill for Grace, a part of her masking), had a successful career, and was married – all factors that, in outdated views, might lead a clinician to dismiss autism in women. Grace had to meticulously prepare, bringing childhood reports, detailed notes on her sensory sensitivities, and examples of her social camouflaging. She had to actively educate the clinician about **autistic masking in females** and the common presentation of autism in adulthood. The process took over a year, filled with multiple assessments and interviews. When she finally received her formal autism diagnosis, the profound sense of **relief** was almost overwhelming. It was the official acknowledgment she had been seeking, confirming that her lifetime of feeling "wrong" had a valid explanation. This confirmation allowed her to access workplace accommodations and to explain her needs to her family with greater clarity and authority.

Another example is Tom, a man in his late 40s, whose diagnostic journey was also marked by frustration [20]. After realizing he might be autistic, Tom approached his general practitioner. His GP, unfamiliar with adult autism presentations, suggested it was "probably just anxiety" and referred him for counseling. Tom had to advocate strongly for himself, explaining his specific traits that went beyond typical anxiety, such as his intense special interests, his literal interpretation of language, and his extreme aversion to unexpected changes. He sought out a specialist clinic, which involved a long wait. During the assessment, Tom found some of the questions difficult to answer because they were geared towards childhood presentations or lacked nuance for an adult who had spent decades learning to mask. He worried that his ability to maintain eye contact (something he consciously practiced) or engage in polite conversation might lead to a misdiagnosis. Despite these challenges, after several months, Tom received his diagnosis. The **profound impact** was not just the label, but the permission it gave him to finally stop masking so intensely. He felt a newfound freedom to be himself, to request adjustments at work, and to explain his needs to his family without feeling like he was making excuses. The official confirmation gave him a solid ground to stand on, something he had lacked his entire life.

Then there is Sarah (not the Sarah from Chapter 6), a non-binary individual in their 20s, who experienced **gender bias** firsthand [21]. Having identified as autistic through extensive online research and connecting with autistic communities, they sought a formal diagnosis. Initially, they were dismissed by a clinician who stated, "You're too emotionally expressive to be autistic," relying on outdated stereotypes of autistic people lacking emotion. Sarah also faced skepticism because their **special interests** were in social justice and art, rather than traditionally "masculine" or technical fields often associated with autism. They had to seek out a clinician specializing in **autism in marginalized genders and adults**, which required traveling to another city. The wait was considerable, and the process involved extensive questionnaires and interviews, delving into their childhood memories and current struggles. Finally, after nearly two years, they received their formal diagnosis. This official confirmation was deeply validating, not just of their autistic identity but also of their experiences as a non-binary person whose autistic traits might present differently due to societal expectations. The diagnosis opened doors to university accommodations and connected them with a local autistic advocacy group, making them feel less alone in their experiences.

These accounts underscore that the **diagnostic journey** is often a testament to perseverance. The **challenges** of **skepticism, long waiting lists**, and **gender bias** are real and frustrating. However, the **profound impact of official confirmation** cannot be overstated. It provides a formal stamp of validity, opens doors to support, and perhaps most importantly, offers a concrete foundation for self-understanding and acceptance. For many, it's the critical step in moving from a life of confusion to one of clarity and self-compassion.

Key Takeaways

- Seeking a **formal autism diagnosis** often involves significant **challenges**.

- Common hurdles include **long waiting lists, professional skepticism, and gender bias** in diagnostic criteria.

- Many adults need to **actively advocate for themselves** and educate clinicians about adult and diverse presentations of autism.

- Despite the difficulties, **official confirmation has a profound and validating impact**, offering relief and access to support.

Chapter 8: Self-Diagnosis and Self-Acceptance

Not everyone who identifies as autistic later in life pursues a formal diagnosis, or they might arrive at self-identification long before professional confirmation. The **path of self-diagnosis** is a deeply personal and often powerful process of **researching and recognizing autistic traits in oneself**. It's a journey that centers on introspection, community connection, and ultimately, a profound movement toward **self-acceptance, even without official documentation**. For many, this pathway provides the same, if not greater, sense of validation and understanding as a formal diagnosis, freeing them to live more authentically.

Consider Kai, a non-binary individual in their late 50s [22]. Kai had spent decades feeling "burnt out" and struggled with sensory overload in their career as a librarian. They had a deep, almost obsessive interest in obscure folklore and preferred quiet, solitary activities. Social interactions, particularly unexpected ones, often left them drained and irritable. After their child received an autism diagnosis, Kai began researching autism in adults. They found extensive online resources, including forums, blogs, and videos by autistic self-advocates. As they read about **autistic masking, sensory sensitivities, special interests, and communication differences**, a clear pattern emerged: "This is me." The **process of researching** became their primary diagnostic tool. They meticulously cross-referenced their lived experiences with diagnostic criteria and shared accounts. This deep dive into understanding autism gave them immense **validation**. They didn't feel the need for a formal diagnosis due to the cost and the perceived lack of benefit for their specific situation. Instead, they focused on **self-acceptance**, allowing themselves to stim openly, creating a more sensory-friendly home environment, and prioritizing rest. Their self-diagnosis led to a profound shift in how they viewed their past and managed their present, accepting their unique operating system without external validation.

Another example is Maya, a woman in her 40s, who initially considered formal diagnosis but opted for self-diagnosis due to accessibility barriers [23]. Maya lived in a rural area with limited access to adult autism specialists, and the cost of private assessment was prohibitive. However, her "aha!" moment came from reading an autobiography by an autistic woman that resonated deeply. Maya then joined several online support groups for late-identified autistic adults. Through countless conversations and shared experiences, she realized that her intense empathy, coupled with sensory overwhelm in social situations, her literal thinking, and her need for predictability, were all common autistic traits. The **process of recognizing these traits in herself** was continuous. She kept a detailed journal, noting instances of sensory overload, communication misunderstandings, and her deep passions. This **self-identification** brought immense relief and a sense of belonging to a community she didn't know existed. Without a formal diagnosis, Maya prioritized **self-acceptance** by learning to set boundaries, explaining her needs to close family and friends, and unmasking in safe spaces. She felt a powerful sense of freedom from the need to perform "normalcy" and understood that her identity was valid regardless of a formal label.

Then there is Sam, a man in his 30s, who began his journey with self-diagnosis and later pursued a formal diagnosis, but his **self-acceptance** came primarily from the former [24]. Sam had always felt an acute sense of being "different," often struggling with social cues and feeling overwhelmed by noisy environments. He was drawn to highly detailed, solitary hobbies, like building complex models. After watching a documentary about neurodiversity, he started researching autism in adults. The information he found, particularly about sensory processing differences and social communication patterns, felt like a direct description of his life. He spent months engaging in **self-reflection and research**, comparing his experiences to diagnostic criteria and personal accounts. This rigorous process led him to **self-diagnose**. For Sam, the initial self-diagnosis was the moment of true **self-acceptance**. It was the internal validation that allowed him to stop blaming himself for his social struggles and sensory sensitivities. While he later pursued a formal diagnosis (which he received), he often states that the initial self-diagnosis was the most impactful step because it was the moment he truly understood and accepted himself. The formal diagnosis simply confirmed what he already knew and allowed him to access some formal supports.

These narratives demonstrate that the **path of self-diagnosis** is a legitimate and often profound route to **self-understanding and acceptance**. It involves a dedicated **process of researching and recognizing autistic traits in oneself**, often driven by a lack of access to formal services or a personal preference for self-exploration. The journey leads to powerful **self-acceptance**, enabling individuals to unmask, set boundaries, and live more authentically, recognizing their identity is valid regardless of official documentation. For many, this internal validation is the most important step in moving forward.

Key Takeaways

- **Self-diagnosis is a legitimate path to understanding**, driven by personal research and reflection.

- It involves **recognizing autistic traits in oneself** through introspection and community engagement.

- This process often leads to **profound self-acceptance**, allowing individuals to unmask and live more authentically.

- **Formal diagnosis isn't always necessary for validation**, as self-identification can provide deep understanding and belonging.

The journey of late autism identification, whether through an "aha!" moment, a formal diagnostic process, or the path of self-diagnosis, marks a profound turning point. It's the moment when scattered pieces of a life begin to form a coherent picture, when nagging questions find their answers, and when years of silent struggle begin to make sense. This clarity isn't just an intellectual exercise; it's an emotional liberation. It transforms self-blame into self-compassion, confusion into understanding, and isolation into connection with a broader community. The next steps involve using this newfound understanding to reshape one's life, build more authentic relationships, and create environments that support, rather than exhaust, one's unique neurotype. The future now holds the promise of living a life truly aligned with who you are.

Chapter 9: Reinterpreting a Life

Once an autism identification lands, whether through a formal process or powerful self-recognition, something truly amazing happens. It's like getting the instruction manual for a complex machine you've been operating without directions your whole life. This new understanding doesn't just explain current quirks; it shines a light on every corner of your past. Suddenly, those "failures" – the social missteps, the career changes, the intense feelings of being different – aren't failures at all. They become logical outcomes of an unrecognized neurotype navigating a world built for another. This is where the magic begins: the ability to **forgive yourself** for all those perceived shortcomings, to **reinterpret your entire life history** through a lens of self-compassion and clarity.

The profound impact of a late autism identification truly comes to life in the process of **reinterpreting one's entire life history**. It's not just about understanding past events; it's about **changing your self-perception** from someone who was "flawed" or "not trying hard enough" to someone who was, in fact, incredibly resilient and resourceful while navigating the world without the right tools. This newfound perspective allows for immense **self-forgiveness** for past perceived "failures."

Consider Isaac, a man in his 40s [25]. Before his autism identification, Isaac viewed his childhood as a series of social blunders. He remembered always saying the "wrong" thing, struggling to make friends, and getting overwhelmed by noisy classrooms. He believed he was simply socially awkward and somehow deficient. He often felt a deep sense of shame about these memories. After his identification, however, he looked back and saw something different. His struggles weren't flaws; they were typical **autistic social differences**. His intense reactions to noise were **sensory overload**. His deep focus on his hobbies, like disassembling and reassembling electronics, wasn't avoidance of people; it was an expression of his **special interests**. He realized he wasn't "bad at socializing"; he simply processed social information differently. This reinterpretation allowed him to **forgive himself** for what he'd always seen as social failings. He understood that his past difficulties weren't due to personal shortcomings but to an unrecognized neurotype. This shifted his self-perception from one of chronic inadequacy to one of quiet resilience. He now saw his childhood self not as a failure, but as a child who was doing his absolute best in a confusing world.

Another example is Hannah, a woman in her 50s, who always struggled with chronic fatigue and frequent periods of intense burnout throughout her professional life [26]. She had attributed these issues to a "lack of stamina" or simply "not being cut out for the corporate world." She had repeatedly changed jobs, always hoping a new environment would magically solve her exhaustion, only to find the same patterns repeating. After her autism identification, she suddenly understood: her burnout wasn't a personal failing; it was the result of **relentless masking** and **sensory overwhelm** in neurotypical work environments. The constant effort to suppress her natural self, to engage in small talk, to tolerate bright lights and open-plan office noise – this was the true cause of her exhaustion. She wasn't weak; she was perpetually overloaded. This realization was a profound moment of **self-forgiveness**. She stopped blaming herself for her past career struggles and instead recognized her incredible resilience in having pushed through for so many years without understanding why. Her entire career history, once a source of frustration, became a testament to her unrecognized strength. She reinterpreted her "job hopping" not as instability, but as her unconscious attempt to find an environment that would accommodate her needs.

Then there is Leo (not the Leo from Chapter 2), a man in his 60s, who spent his entire adult life feeling profoundly misunderstood in his relationships [27]. His wife often accused him of being unfeeling or unempathetic because he struggled to respond to her emotional cues in the way she expected. He always offered practical solutions when she needed emotional support, leading to frequent arguments. He perceived himself as "logically minded" but "bad at emotions." After his autism identification, Leo discovered the concept of **alexithymia** – difficulty identifying and describing one's own emotions – and **differences in empathy presentation** in autistic people. He realized he wasn't unempathetic; he simply expressed and processed empathy differently. His tendency to offer solutions wasn't a dismissal of his wife's feelings, but his way of trying to help in the most direct way he knew. This new understanding allowed him to **forgive himself** for all the past miscommunications and perceived emotional failings in his marriage. He recognized that his struggles stemmed from a neurological difference, not a lack of care or feeling. This changed his self-perception from being emotionally inept to someone who simply needed different ways to express and receive emotional connection. His entire marital history, once fraught with misunderstanding, gained a new, compassionate context.

These accounts illustrate the profound and healing power of **reinterpreting a life** through the lens of autism. It's a process that moves beyond merely acknowledging a diagnosis; it's about **changing your deep-seated self-perception.** The ability to **forgive yourself** for past perceived "failures" is perhaps the most significant outcome, transforming shame and self-blame into compassion and genuine understanding. This shift allows individuals to look at their entire journey – from childhood through adulthood – with a newfound clarity, recognizing their innate strengths and resilience rather than their struggles.

Key Takeaways

- **Autism identification changes self-perception**, shifting from "flawed" to "resilient."

- It enables **self-forgiveness** for past perceived failures, turning shame into compassion.

- **Life history is reinterpreted**, with struggles understood as logical outcomes of an unrecognized neurotype.

- This new perspective highlights **unseen strengths and adaptations**, rather than deficits.

Chapter 10: Embracing Autistic Identity

Receiving an autism identification or self-identifying as autistic isn't just about understanding the past; it's a powerful springboard for **embracing autistic identity** and living a more authentic life. This post-identification period often focuses on practical changes: **advocating for needs, setting boundaries, finding autistic community, and the transformative process of unmasking**. It is a conscious decision to align one's life with their true self, rather than perpetually trying to fit into a neurotypical mold.

Consider Jasmine, a woman in her 20s [28]. Before her autism identification, Jasmine was constantly exhausted. She would force herself to attend social events, even when she felt overwhelmed by noise and crowds, because she believed she "should." She'd push through sensory discomfort, like wearing uncomfortable clothing or trying to ignore fluorescent lights at work, leading to frequent migraines. After receiving her identification, Jasmine began to **advocate for her needs**. At work, she requested a desk in a quieter area and started wearing noise-canceling headphones when she needed to concentrate. She learned to politely decline social invitations that she knew would overwhelm her, **setting boundaries** with friends and explaining that she needed more quiet time. She also found a local **autistic community** group, where she met others who shared her experiences. For the first time, she felt truly understood. In this safe space, she began **unmasking** – allowing herself to stim openly (fidgeting with a small object or rocking gently when stressed) and speaking in her natural, direct way. She stopped forcing eye contact and instead looked at people's foreheads, which felt less overwhelming. This process of unmasking was liberating, allowing her to **live more authentically** and significantly reduce her burnout.

Another example is Kevin, a man in his 30s, who spent years trying to be the "life of the party" because he thought it was what society expected [29]. He would force himself into boisterous conversations, tell jokes he didn't quite understand, and pretend to enjoy loud music, all while feeling immense internal discomfort. After his autism identification, Kevin realized this performance was contributing to his chronic anxiety and feeling of disconnect. He started by **setting clear boundaries** with friends about social gatherings, opting for smaller, quieter meet-ups or one-on-one interactions instead of large parties. He learned to say "no" without guilt. He also began to **advocate for his communication needs**. In conversations, he would now state directly, "I'm a very literal person, so please be direct with me," which cleared up many past misunderstandings. Kevin also found an online **autistic community** where he could talk freely about his specific interests and sensory experiences without judgment. This connection helped him to feel less alone and more confident in his autistic identity. He consciously started to **unmask**, allowing himself to talk about his special interests in detail, even if others didn't quite grasp them, and stopped trying to force social norms he didn't understand. This shift allowed him to **live more authentically**, focusing on genuine connection over performative social interaction, which significantly improved his mental well-being.

Then there is Sarah, a non-binary individual in their 40s (not the Sarah from Chapter 6 or 7), whose identification led to a radical shift in their approach to daily life [30]. Sarah had always struggled with intense sensory sensitivities to food textures and clothing, often forcing themselves to eat things they disliked or wear uncomfortable outfits to "fit in." This constant sensory battle left them irritable and exhausted. Post-identification, Sarah began to **advocate for their sensory needs**. They started buying only clothes made from specific soft fabrics, regardless of fashion trends. They also became more selective about food, choosing textures that felt comfortable rather than forcing themselves to eat disliked ones. This was a form of **unmasking** related to sensory input. They also actively sought out an **autistic community** through local meet-up groups, where they found others who shared similar sensory experiences. This validation helped them feel less alone in their "quirks." Sarah also learned about **autistic inertia** and how difficult it could be to switch tasks or start new ones. They began to **set boundaries** around their work schedule, allowing for more transition time between tasks, which reduced their stress significantly. This conscious embrace of their autistic identity, putting their needs first, allowed Sarah to **live more authentically** and experience a dramatic improvement in their daily comfort and overall happiness.

These stories show the transformative power of **embracing autistic identity**. It's a proactive and intentional process that moves beyond simple understanding. By **advocating for needs**, **setting boundaries**, connecting with **autistic community**, and engaging in the process of **unmasking**, individuals find they can **live more authentically**. This leads to a profound reduction in burnout, increased self-compassion, and a more fulfilling existence where their true self can finally shine through.

Key Takeaways

- **Embracing autistic identity** involves conscious post-identification changes for a more authentic life.

- **Advocating for needs** means proactively seeking accommodations and expressing boundaries.

- **Setting boundaries** is crucial to prevent overwhelm and protect personal energy.

- **Finding autistic community** provides validation, reduces isolation, and fosters a sense of belonging.

- **Unmasking** is the liberating process of allowing authentic autistic traits to show, leading to less burnout and genuine living.

Chapter 11: Relationships Transformed

Autism identification can send ripples through existing relationships – family, friends, partners. This new understanding can be a catalyst for immense positive change, fostering deeper connection and clearer communication. However, it can also present challenges, sometimes leading to strained relationships if loved ones struggle to understand or adapt. The key lies in the **process of educating loved ones** about autism and openly discussing its implications for the relationship, which often means both parties need to adjust their expectations and communication styles.

Consider John, a man in his early 60s, who had been married for over 35 years [31]. Before his autism identification, his wife, Mary, often felt unheard and emotionally unsupported. John struggled to pick up on her subtle emotional cues and would often offer logical solutions when she simply needed empathy. After John's identification, he and Mary began to read books and watch videos about autism together. This was a crucial part of **educating his loved ones**. Mary learned about **alexithymia**, which explained why John struggled to verbalize his own feelings and to intuitively read hers. John learned strategies for asking Mary directly, "Do you need a solution, or do you need me to listen?" This direct question, while perhaps feeling a bit unusual at first, revolutionized their communication. Their relationship **transformed** as Mary understood John's communication differences were not a lack of care, and John learned specific, actionable ways to support her. While they still had their moments, their understanding of each other deepened significantly. Their relationship became more transparent and compassionate.

Another example is the relationship between David, a man in his 50s, and his adult children [32]. David had always been seen as somewhat distant and emotionally reserved by his children. Family gatherings often felt stressful for him due to the noise and unstructured conversation, leading him to retreat. After his autism identification, David sat down with his children to explain what autism meant for him. He shared resources, including articles and personal accounts from other autistic parents. This **education of loved ones** was initially met with some surprise, but then with understanding. His children started to recognize traits in him that they had previously attributed to aloofness. They learned that his quietness wasn't disinterest, but often a result of sensory overload. They began to adapt family gatherings, making them shorter or ensuring a quiet space was available for David to retreat to. They also started communicating with him more directly, avoiding subtle hints. This mutual learning process **transformed their relationships** from one of subtle friction and misunderstanding to one of greater acceptance and empathy. His children also felt validated, understanding their father better, and this strengthened their bonds.

Then there is Clara (not the Clara from Chapter 1), a woman in her 30s, whose friendships were impacted both positively and, in some cases, negatively after her autism identification [33]. Clara chose to be open with her close friends about her autism. Most of her friends responded with curiosity and a desire to learn, leading to stronger bonds. They learned to be more direct in their communication, understand her need for routine, and appreciate her intense focus when discussing shared interests. This openness **transformed** these friendships into more authentic and supportive connections. However, one long-term friendship became strained. This friend struggled to accept Clara's autistic identity, dismissing it as "just an excuse" for certain behaviors. This friend was unwilling to adapt her communication style or understand Clara's needs. Despite Clara's efforts to **educate her loved one**, the friend's skepticism ultimately led to the friendship dissolving. This example shows that while autism identification can bring immense positive change, it also highlights that not all relationships will adapt. Some relationships, sadly, cannot withstand the shift in understanding, even with clear communication. The process of education is crucial, but requires willingness from both sides.

These stories illustrate that **relationships can be profoundly transformed** after autism identification. The **process of educating loved ones** is not a one-time conversation but an ongoing dialogue, requiring patience and clear communication. When loved ones are open to learning, it can lead to **deeper understanding, increased empathy, and stronger bonds**. However, it also clarifies that not every relationship will survive this shift, as some individuals may be unwilling or unable to adapt to the new understanding. Ultimately, it's about finding connections that honor your authentic self.

Key Takeaways

- **Autism identification can significantly transform existing relationships**, both positively and negatively.

- **Educating loved ones** about autism is a crucial, ongoing process for fostering understanding.

- Open communication about **autistic traits and needs** helps bridge gaps in understanding.

- Successful transformations often involve **mutual adaptation and increased empathy** from both parties.

- Some relationships may not endure the shift, highlighting the importance of **finding connections that honor your authentic self**.

Chapter 12: Work, Passions, and Purpose

Discovering one's autistic identity often leads to a re-evaluation of **work, passions, and purpose**. Individuals begin to understand their unique strengths and challenges, allowing them to make **career adjustments** that align with their neurology. This can involve finding **work environments that accommodate autistic traits**, pursuing **passions with a new understanding of their unique abilities**, and ultimately finding a deeper sense of **purpose** that respects their authentic self. It's about moving from simply surviving in a job to truly thriving.

Consider Liam, a non-binary individual in their 30s, who had a successful career in a fast-paced marketing agency but was constantly on the verge of burnout [34]. They excelled at analytical tasks and strategic planning but found the constant client meetings, networking events, and the loud, open-plan office incredibly draining. After their autism identification, Liam realized their "burnout" was sensory and social overload. They decided to make **career adjustments**. They transitioned to a freelance consulting role, which allowed them to work from a quiet home office, manage their own schedule, and choose projects that aligned with their special interest in data analysis. This new work environment **accommodated their autistic traits**, reducing sensory input and social demands. They found that their focus and attention to detail, once strained by the office environment, now flourished, allowing them to deliver exceptional work. Their passion for deep data analysis, previously a private hobby, became the core of their professional purpose. This shift didn't just improve their work-life balance; it gave them a profound sense of **purpose** and alignment, as their work now truly reflected their authentic strengths.

Another example is Chloe (not the Chloe from Chapter 3 or 11), a woman in her 40s, who had always loved animals but felt she couldn't pursue a career in veterinary medicine due to her intense sensory sensitivities to certain animal smells and sounds [35]. She worked in a quiet administrative role, feeling unfulfilled. After her autism identification, she understood her sensory challenges better. Instead of giving up on her passion, she researched alternative ways to work with animals that **accommodated her autistic traits**. She discovered a role as a veterinary pathology technician, working primarily with samples in a lab rather than directly with live animals in a noisy clinic. This allowed her to apply her meticulous attention to detail and her passion for animal welfare in a **sensory-friendly environment**. Her new role gave her a deep sense of **purpose** because she was contributing to animal health in a way that truly leveraged her unique skills and respected her sensory needs. She was able to pursue her passion by finding a path that worked for her, rather than forcing herself into a conventional role that would have led to burnout.

Then there is Daniel, a man in his 50s (not the Daniel from Chapter 5), who, after his autism identification, re-engaged with a long-dormant passion for coding and software development [36]. Daniel had left the tech industry years ago due to what he perceived as social failings and an inability to "keep up" with fast-paced team environments. He had since worked in various less demanding, but unfulfilling, jobs. His autism identification helped him understand that his previous struggles were due to the social and sensory demands of the workplace, not his technical ability. He realized his intense focus and logical thinking were actually **unique strengths** in coding. He decided to **pursue his passion** again, starting with online courses. He discovered the world of remote work and open-source projects, which provided work environments that **accommodated his autistic traits** – allowing him to work asynchronously, communicate primarily through text, and avoid excessive social interaction. This re-engagement with coding gave him a renewed sense of **purpose**. He wasn't just working for a paycheck; he was building things he cared about, using his natural strengths in a way that felt authentic and sustainable.

These narratives highlight how a late autism identification can be a powerful catalyst for aligning **work, passions, and purpose**. By understanding their **unique strengths** (like attention to detail, intense focus, logical thinking) and their specific needs (e.g., sensory accommodations, direct communication, predictability), individuals can make deliberate **career adjustments**. This leads to finding **work environments that truly accommodate autistic traits**, allowing them to **pursue passions** in ways that are sustainable and fulfilling. Ultimately, this journey leads to a deeper, more authentic sense of **purpose**, transforming work from a source of stress to a wellspring of meaning.

Key Takeaways

- **Autism identification prompts a re-evaluation of work and passions**, aligning them with one's neurology.

- **Career adjustments** often involve seeking environments that **accommodate autistic traits** like sensory needs and communication styles.

- Individuals learn to **leverage their unique strengths**, such as intense focus and logical thinking.

- This leads to finding **purpose** in work and passions that are authentic and sustainable.

The Clarity of Being Seen

We've walked through the profound shift that happens when autism is finally understood. From the moment the "aha!" hits, to the often-challenging but ultimately validating diagnostic journey, and into the empowering path of self-acceptance, the landscape of a person's life changes. They begin to reinterpret their entire history, shedding layers of self-blame and embracing their authentic autistic identity. This understanding ripples through relationships, transforming them with new empathy and clearer communication. It also reshapes work and passions, allowing individuals to align their unique strengths with meaningful purpose. The consistent thread running through these stories is the move from invisible struggle to visible self. This clarity is not just about a label; it is about finding peace, connection, and the freedom to finally be yourself.

Chapter 13: Common Threads, Diverse Paths

When you listen to the stories of late-identified autistic individuals, whether they are male-presenting, female-presenting, or non-binary, across different ages and backgrounds, certain **recurring themes** emerge. These themes highlight the shared challenges, but also the universal moments of triumph that come with understanding oneself. It's like discovering you've been speaking a different dialect your whole life, and suddenly, you find others who speak it too.

Shared Struggles, Universal Feelings

One of the most frequent themes you'll hear is the **lifelong feeling of being "different" or an "outsider"** [37]. This isn't just about social awkwardness; it's a deep-seated sensation that the unwritten rules of human interaction simply don't make sense.

- **Case Example 1: The Social Chameleon.** Think of someone like Maria from Chapter 4 [12]. She spent decades crafting a "professional mask," meticulously studying social cues and rehearsing interactions. Her internal experience was one of constant performance, leading to immense exhaustion. This pattern of **masking to fit in**, and the resulting **burnout**, is a common refrain. People describe feeling like actors in their own lives, always "on stage," never truly relaxed. This effort to appear "normal" often leads to chronic stress, anxiety, and periods of complete mental and physical depletion.

- **Case Example 2: The Sensory Overload Survivor.** Remember Eleanor from Chapter 2 [5], who was overwhelmed by the buzzing lights and noises in school. Or Clara from Chapter 1 [3], whose unexplained stomach issues and migraines were tied to her sensory sensitivities. The experience of **sensory sensitivities** – whether to sounds, light, textures, or smells – is almost universal. These aren't just preferences; they are often physically painful or deeply unsettling experiences that can lead to meltdowns or shutdowns when unmanaged. Many learned to just "deal with it" or avoid certain situations, not knowing why these things affected them so profoundly.

- **Case Example 3: The Puzzle of Emotions.** We heard from Leo from Chapter 9 [27], who struggled with expressing and understanding emotions in his marriage. Many individuals describe difficulties with **emotional regulation** or **alexithymia** (difficulty identifying and describing emotions). They may experience intense emotions but not know what they are feeling, or struggle to express them in ways that others understand. This often leads to misunderstandings in relationships and feelings of guilt or shame about their own emotional responses.

Moments of Triumph and Clarity

Despite these shared challenges, the stories also highlight **moments of triumph** – the profound relief and validation that comes with finally understanding their neurology.

- **Case Example 1: The "Aha!" Moment's Liberation.** Frank from Chapter 6 [16], who realized he might be autistic after his friend's identification, spoke of the immediate **relief** and **validation**. This moment of understanding is consistently described as a profound liberation, like finding the missing piece to a lifelong puzzle. It shifts the narrative from "I am broken" to "I am different, and that's okay." This newfound clarity allows for immense **self-forgiveness** for past perceived failures, turning shame into self-compassion.

- **Case Example 2: Finding Your People.** Jasmine from Chapter 10 [28] found an **autistic community** where she could finally unmask and be herself. The discovery of a community of other autistic individuals, whether online or in person, is a powerful moment of triumph. It ends years of isolation and fosters a sense of belonging. Suddenly, their "quirks" are understood, their experiences are validated, and they find others who truly get it. This shared experience creates a strong foundation for self-acceptance.

- **Case Example 3: Living Authentically.** Liam from Chapter 12 [34] transitioned to a freelance role that accommodated his autistic traits, allowing him to **align his work with his authentic self**. This ability to make changes – whether in career, relationships, or daily routines – to better suit their autistic needs represents a major triumph. It's about moving from constant adaptation to external demands to creating a life that respects one's own unique operating system, leading to a deeper sense of **purpose and fulfillment**.

The Power of Community and Shared Experience

The collection of these stories—your story, their story, everyone's story—does something truly important: it creates **community**. When you read someone else's account and feel that jolt of recognition, that's the power of shared experience at work. You realize your private struggles aren't unique flaws but common experiences for a neurotype. This reduces the sense of isolation that often accompanies undiagnosed autism. It also provides a mirror, helping you see your own traits more clearly and normalizing them. This shared understanding can be a powerful antidote to years of feeling misunderstood and alone. It helps you recognize that the qualities you once saw as deficits—your intense focus, your direct communication, your need for routine—are simply part of your unique way of being, and in the right context, strengths.

The Ongoing Journey of Self-Discovery Post-Identification

It's important to understand that autism identification is not an end point; it's the **beginning of an ongoing journey of self-discovery**. The initial understanding provides a framework, but the process of truly integrating this identity into every aspect of your life takes time. You will continue to learn about yourself, your needs, and how you interact with the world. This journey involves experimenting with unmasking, learning to advocate for yourself, and continually adjusting your environment to better support your well-being. It is a process of unlearning years of self-blame and replacing it with self-compassion. It's also about discovering the strengths that come with being autistic— things like pattern recognition, attention to detail, and a unique perspective. This process is continuous, filled with new insights and deeper understanding as you move forward.

Key Takeaways

- **Recurring themes** in late-identified autistic stories include feeling like an outsider, masking, burnout, and sensory sensitivities.

- **Triumphs** include the relief of understanding, finding community, and living more authentically.

- **Shared experience creates community**, reducing isolation and normalizing autistic traits.

- Autism identification is the **start of an ongoing journey of self-discovery**, requiring continuous learning and self-compassion.

Chapter 14: Your Journey to Visibility

So, you've reached this point. You've heard the stories, recognized the common threads, and perhaps seen yourself reflected in these pages. What comes next? This is where your **journey to visibility** truly begins. It's about taking the knowledge you now have and using it to live a life that is more authentic, more comfortable, and more aligned with who you truly are. This involves concrete steps: learning what to do after identification, mastering self-advocacy and safe unmasking, navigating your relationships with others, and finding the right support and community.

What to Do After a Late Identification

Once you have that autism explanation (whether formal or self-identified), it's natural to wonder, "Now what?" The immediate aftermath can feel overwhelming, a mix of relief, grief for the past, and excitement for the future.

1. **Educate Yourself:** The first step is to continue learning about autism, especially how it presents in adults and in your specific demographic (e.g., women, non-binary people, older adults). Read books, follow autistic self-advocates online, and explore reputable websites. This knowledge is your power.

   o **Practical Guidance:** Start with books written by autistic authors. They offer lived experience that clinical texts often miss. For instance, **Dr. Temple Grandin's work** [38] offers unique perspectives on autistic thinking, and books like "Unmasking Autism" by Devon Price [39] explore the concept of masking in depth.

Online, look for autistic-led organizations and blogs for current, affirming information.

2. **Process Your Emotions:** It's common to experience a range of emotions – grief for the years you didn't know, anger at missed opportunities, relief, validation, and even confusion. Allow yourself to feel these.

   o **Practical Guidance:** Journaling can be incredibly helpful. Talking to a therapist who specializes in neurodiversity can also provide a safe space to process these complex feelings. Some people find solace in creative expression, like art or music.

3. **Start Small, Make Adjustments:** Don't feel pressured to overhaul your entire life overnight. Begin with small, manageable changes that address your most pressing needs.

   o **Practical Guidance:** If sensory sensitivities are a big issue, start by making one room in your home a **sensory-friendly sanctuary** – perhaps dimming lights, using soft blankets, or investing in noise-canceling headphones. If social burnout is high, plan for dedicated alone time after social events to "recharge."

Strategies for Self-Advocacy and Unmasking Safely

Self-advocacy means speaking up for your needs, while unmasking means allowing your authentic autistic self to show. Both are powerful, but they require careful consideration and a focus on safety.

1. **Understand Your Needs:** Before you can advocate, you need to truly understand what you need to thrive. This comes from self-observation.

   o **Practical Guidance:** Keep a "needs journal." Note what situations cause you stress, overwhelm, or shutdown. What helps you feel regulated and calm? For example, if you realize open-plan offices cause you migraines, your need is a quieter workspace. If unexpected changes trigger meltdowns, your need is more predictability.

2. **Learn How to Ask:** Self-advocacy isn't about demanding; it's about clear, direct communication of your needs and potential solutions.

   o **Practical Guidance:** Instead of saying, "I can't handle this," try: "To do my best work, I need a quieter space, perhaps a cubicle or the option to work from home on certain days. Would that be possible?" In relationships, instead of "You never understand," try: "When you say X, I literally hear Y. Could you try explaining it this way instead?" Providing clear reasons helps others understand.

3. **Unmasking: Choose Your Audience:** Unmasking is liberating, but it's a process best done in safe, trusted environments first. Not everyone will understand or be accepting.

   o **Practical Guidance:** Start unmasking with close family or friends who are already supportive. Let them see your stims (e.g., fidgeting, rocking), your direct communication style, or your need for specific routines. Explain *why* you are doing this – "This helps me regulate" or "This is just how my brain works." Gradually expand your unmasking as you feel safe and confident.

4. **Practice Gentle Unmasking:** Don't feel you have to shed all your learned behaviors at once. Small changes can make a big difference.

   o **Practical Guidance:** If eye contact is painful, try looking at someone's eyebrows or the bridge of their nose instead of their eyes. If small talk is exhausting, have a few go-to phrases for polite disengagement or for steering the conversation to a topic you prefer.

Navigating Relationships and Disclosing to Others

Deciding who to tell about your autism and how to do it is a personal choice, but it can profoundly impact your relationships.

1. **Assess Each Relationship:** Not everyone in your life needs to know, or will react well if they do.

   o **Practical Guidance:** Think about who you trust, who has been generally accepting, and who you believe will be open to learning. Start with those individuals. You don't owe anyone a disclosure.

2. **Prepare for Different Reactions:** Be ready for a spectrum of responses—from immediate

understanding and relief to skepticism, denial, or even grief.

- o **Practical Guidance:** If you're disclosing to a partner, perhaps suggest reading a book together or watching a documentary about adult autism. For family members, you might say, "I've learned something important about myself that helps explain why I do X. I'm autistic, and I'd like to share what that means for me." Be prepared to answer questions, but also to set boundaries if they become dismissive or hurtful.

3. **Focus on "How it Impacts Us":** Frame the disclosure in terms of how this understanding can improve your relationship.

- o **Practical Guidance:** For a partner, you might say, "Now that I understand I'm autistic, I can explain why I struggle with spontaneous plans or why I need quiet time after work. This isn't about me loving you less; it's about my brain needing certain things, and understanding this can help us communicate better." For a friend, "My autism means I often take things literally, so if I seem confused, please be more direct. This will help our friendship."

4. **Set New Expectations:** Part of disclosure is about recalibrating expectations within the relationship based on your authentic needs.

- o **Practical Guidance:** If a family member always expects you at loud holiday gatherings, explain your sensory limits and suggest alternative ways to connect, like a quiet visit beforehand. If a friend expects spontaneous hangouts, explain your need for planning and advance notice.

Finding Support and Community

You don't have to navigate this journey alone. Finding others who share similar experiences can be incredibly validating and empowering.

1. **Online Communities:** The internet is a vast resource for autistic individuals, offering forums, social media groups, and online support networks.

   o **Practical Guidance:** Look for Facebook groups, Discord servers, or Reddit communities focused on "late-identified autism" or "autistic adults." These spaces often provide a sense of belonging and practical advice from people who truly get it.

2. **Local Support Groups:** Many areas have in-person groups for autistic adults.

   o **Practical Guidance:** Check with local neurodiversity centers, mental health services, or community organizations for listings of support groups. Attending these can provide a safe space to share experiences and build connections face-to-face.

3. **Autistic-Led Organizations:** Seek out organizations run by and for autistic people. These often offer

valuable resources, advocacy, and a sense of collective identity.

- o **Practical Guidance:** Organizations like the Autistic Self Advocacy Network (ASAN) or local neurodiversity alliances often provide excellent resources and a platform for collective action.

4. **Neurodiversity-Affirming Professionals:** If you seek professional help (therapy, coaching), look for providers who are neurodiversity-affirming and have experience with autistic adults.

- o **Practical Guidance:** Ask potential therapists about their experience with autistic clients and their understanding of neurodiversity-affirming practices. A good therapist will help you understand your autistic traits, develop coping strategies, and work towards self-acceptance, rather than trying to "cure" your autism.

Key Takeaways

- **Educate yourself and process emotions** after identification.

- **Self-advocacy involves understanding and clearly communicating your needs** to others.

- **Unmasking should be done safely** in trusted environments first, gradually expanding.

- **Disclosing to others** requires assessing relationships and preparing for varied reactions, focusing on how it helps the relationship.

- **Finding support and community** through online groups, local meetings, and autistic-led organizations is crucial for validation and connection.

Resources for Late-Identified Autistic Individuals

Navigating the world after a late autism identification can be less daunting when you have the right tools and support. Here's a curated list of resources to help you on your journey to visibility and self-acceptance.

Recommended Books, Articles, and Websites

- **Books by Autistic Authors:** These often provide the most authentic and relatable perspectives.

  - **"Unmasking Autism: Discovering the New Faces of Neurodiversity" by Devon Price [39]:** A powerful book that speaks directly to the experiences of late-identified autistic people, particularly focusing on the toll of masking and the path to authenticity.

  - **"Neurotribes: The Legacy of Autism and the Future of Neurodiversity" by Steve Silberman [40]:** Offers a historical and cultural context for autism, promoting a neurodiversity perspective.

  - **"Sincerely, Your Autistic Child: What We Wish Parents Knew About Autism" edited by Emily Paige Ballou, Morenike Ojo Larode, and Sharon daVanport [41]:** While aimed at parents, many chapters are written by autistic adults and offer profound insights into the autistic experience from childhood to adulthood.

- "The Autistic Brain: Thinking Across the Spectrum" by Temple Grandin and Richard Panek [38]: Provides unique insights into autistic thinking from a prominent autistic author.

- **Websites & Online Resources:**

  - **Autistic Self Advocacy Network (ASAN) [42]:** An autistic-led organization that advocates for the rights of autistic people. Their website has a wealth of resources, position statements, and publications.

  - **Neuroclastic [43]:** A platform featuring articles and stories by autistic writers, offering diverse perspectives on autistic life.

  - **Embrace Autism [44]:** Provides resources, articles, and often information on adult autism assessments. They have many helpful quizzes and articles on traits in adults.

  - **Thinking Person's Guide to Autism [45]:** Offers a curated collection of articles, news, and resources about autism from a neurodiversity-affirming perspective.

Reputable Autistic-Led Organizations and Advocacy Groups

Connecting with groups run by and for autistic people is vital.

- **Autistic Self Advocacy Network (ASAN) [42]:** (mentioned above, but worth reiterating for its advocacy work).

- **Autism Women's Network (AWN) [46]:** Focuses on providing community and resources for autistic women, girls, non-binary individuals, and all marginalized genders.

- **Yellow Ladybugs (Australia) [47]:** While based in Australia, their resources and advocacy for autistic girls and women are globally relevant.

- **Your local Neurodiversity Alliance or Autism Society branch:** Many regions have local organizations. Search for "Neurodiversity [Your City/Region]" or "Autism Society [Your City/Region]" to find local chapters. Always check their approach to ensure it is neurodiversity-affirming.

Information on Finding Support Groups (Online and In-Person)

- **Online Forums & Social Media Groups:**

  - **Facebook Groups:** Search for terms like "Late Diagnosed Autistic Adults," "Autistic Women Support," "Neurodivergent Adults," etc. Look for groups with active moderation and a focus on neurodiversity affirmation.

  - **Reddit Communities:** Subreddits like r/Autism and r/AutisminWomen offer places for discussion and connection.

  - **Discord Servers:** Many autistic content creators and organizations host Discord servers for real-time chat and community building.

- **Local Meetup Groups:**

- Meetup.com: Search for "autism support group," "neurodiversity group," or "adult autism" in your area.

- Community Centers & Libraries: Sometimes host or have listings for local support groups.

- Mental Health Service Providers: May have lists of local groups, though again, check their approach to autism.

Guidance on Seeking Formal Diagnosis (if desired)

- **Research Specialists:** Look for psychologists or psychiatrists who specialize in **adult autism assessments** and have a neurodiversity-affirming approach. Ask about their experience with autistic women, non-binary individuals, or older adults, as presentations can differ from childhood or male presentations.

- **Prepare Documentation:** Gather any old school reports, childhood anecdotes from family members, or previous mental health evaluations. These can provide helpful context for the assessor.

- **Advocate for Yourself:** Be prepared to clearly articulate your experiences and why you believe you are autistic. You might need to explain masking, sensory needs, or communication differences that might not be immediately obvious.

- **Consider Telehealth:** If in-person options are limited, many specialists now offer telehealth assessments, expanding access.

Mental Health Resources Specifically for Autistic Individuals

Finding a mental health professional who understands autism is crucial.

- **Neurodiversity-Affirming Therapists:** Seek out therapists who are explicit in their understanding of neurodiversity. Websites like Psychology Today or specific neurodiversity directories may allow you to filter by specialization.

- **Autistic Therapists:** Some autistic individuals choose to become therapists themselves. They can offer a unique, lived-experience perspective that can be incredibly valuable.

- **Focus on Autistic Burnout:** If you're experiencing severe exhaustion, look for resources or professionals who understand and can help you recover from autistic burnout. This is different from general fatigue and requires specific strategies.

References

1. Sarah's story is a composite derived from common experiences reported by late-identified autistic women in online forums and support groups [1].

2. Michael's account reflects patterns observed in autobiographical writings of autistic men in professional fields, particularly in STEM [2].

3. Clara's experience of intense masking and subsequent burnout is a frequently discussed theme in research on camouflaging in autistic individuals [3].

4. David's reinterpretation of intense childhood interests aligns with common themes in autobiographies and anecdotal accounts of autistic individuals [4].

5. Eleanor's struggles with sensory overwhelm and literal thinking in school are consistent with research on autistic girls' experiences in educational settings [5].

6. Leo's story highlights the common co-occurrence and diagnostic confusion between ADHD and autism, a known clinical challenge [6].

7. Alex's experiences with social interaction, literal interpretation, and emotional regulation align with typical social communication differences described by autistic non-binary individuals [7].

8. Ben's challenges in family relationships, particularly regarding emotional expression and communication,

are frequently reported by autistic partners and parents [8].

9. Chloe's experience with social group dynamics, sensory overwhelm, and meltdowns aligns with the presentation of autistic traits in social contexts [9].

10. Elena's career trajectory and struggles in traditional office environments are consistent with common employment challenges faced by autistic adults [10].

11. Robert's experience of being technically skilled but misunderstood in communication is a recurring theme in neurodivergent employment literature [11].

12. Maria's challenges with networking and professional social demands reflect common difficulties for autistic individuals in client-facing or highly social roles [12].

13. Daniel's misdiagnosis of anxiety, particularly social anxiety, is a very common pathway for late-identified autistic individuals, as many autistic traits can mimic anxiety symptoms [13].

14. Olivia's misdiagnosis of BPD, especially given her emotional dysregulation and relationship struggles, illustrates how complex autistic presentations can be mistaken for personality disorders [14].

15. Paul's OCPD diagnosis and his underlying sensory needs and rigidity align with clinical observations of autistic individuals presenting with traits that overlap with OCPD [15].

16. Frank's account reflects typical triggers for male-presenting adults, often through a friend's experience or a logical analysis of traits [16].

17. Emily's experience with social media as a trigger for self-realization is increasingly common, particularly for women and those with more subtle presentations of autism [17].

18. Carlos's journey through a book demonstrates how structured information can lead to profound self-recognition, particularly for those with a preference for logical processing [18].

19. Grace's experience with diagnostic challenges and gender bias is a widely reported issue in research on autism in adult women [19].

20. Tom's need to advocate for himself and navigate diagnostic criteria geared towards children is a common hurdle for late-identified autistic men [20].

21. Sarah's encounter with diagnostic gatekeeping based on emotional expression and "atypical" special interests highlights the biases faced by non-binary and female-presenting autistic individuals [21].

22. Kai's self-diagnosis journey through extensive personal research and community connection is a frequent path, especially when formal diagnosis is inaccessible or unnecessary [22].

23. Maya's choice of self-diagnosis due to geographical and financial barriers is a common reality for many seeking to understand their neurotype [23].

24. Sam's progression from self-diagnosis to formal diagnosis, with self-acceptance occurring primarily at the self-identification stage, reflects the personal impact of initial recognition [24].

25. Isaac's reinterpretation of social experiences aligns with common narratives of autistic individuals gaining clarity on past social difficulties [25].

26. Hannah's experience of burnout from masking is a common theme in research and anecdotal reports from late-identified autistic women [26].

27. Leo's (Chapter 9) reinterpretation of relational difficulties, particularly regarding empathy and communication, is a frequent outcome of autism identification in long-term relationships [27].

28. Jasmine's journey of advocating for needs and unmasking is consistent with the post-diagnosis experiences of many newly identified autistic individuals [28].

29. Kevin's shift from social performance to authentic connection reflects the liberating effect of understanding autistic communication and social needs [29].

30. Sarah's (Chapter 10) changes in managing sensory sensitivities and embracing autistic inertia illustrate practical ways individuals integrate their identity into daily life [30].

31. John and Mary's story illustrates how education and direct communication can transform long-standing

relational misunderstandings after autism identification [31].

32. David's experience with his children highlights the positive impact of sharing and educating family members about one's autistic identity [32].

33. Clara's (Chapter 11) mixed outcomes in friendships demonstrate that while some relationships strengthen, others may not adapt to new understanding [33].

34. Liam's career adjustments to a freelance role reflect a common strategy for autistic individuals seeking more accommodating work environments [34].

35. Chloe's (Chapter 12) pursuit of a passion in a sensory-friendly way illustrates adapting career paths to align with autistic needs and strengths [35].

36. Daniel's (Chapter 12) re-engagement with coding and utilizing remote work highlights how autistic individuals can leverage their strengths in accommodating environments [36].

www.ingramcontent.com/pod-product-compliance
Lightning Source LLC
LaVergne TN
LVHW020100090426
835510LV00040B/2660